W9-CIR-996

The Art of the IV Start

Testimonial Page

"Although I was taught how to start IVs in nursing school, my success rate prior to receiving Bob's advice was close to 50%. Now....my success rate has jumped to nearly 90%."
                                                          Kati Masters RN

"Due to Bob's advice, I have become one of the *go to* nurses called for starting difficult IVs hospital wide."
                                                          Bill Bricker RN, CCRN

"Bob helped improve my IV skills tremendously. He gave me the confidence to believe I would and could succeed with practice."
                                                          Megan Smith RN

"Since Bob's review of IV skills, my insertion success rate is about 90% on the first stick. Instead of it being a nervous and dreaded task, it has become one I am confident in and actually enjoy doing."
                                                          Renee Saylor RN

The Art of the IV Start

Common Techniques and Tricks of the Trade for Establishing Successful Peripheral Intravenous Lines

Bob Rynecki MS, RN, CCRN-CMC

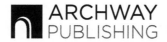

ARCHWAY PUBLISHING

Copyright © 2014 Robert P. Rynecki MS, RN, CCRN-CMC.

All rights reserved. No part of this book may be used or reproduced by any means, graphic, electronic, or mechanical, including photocopying, recording, taping or by any information storage retrieval system without the written permission of the publisher except in the case of brief quotations embodied in critical articles and reviews.

The information, ideas, and suggestions in this book are not intended as a substitute for medical training or the rules and practices of any medical facility. There are no express or implied representations or warranties, including accuracy, compliance with present or future applicable standards of care, or applicability to a particular situation. Neither the author nor the publisher shall be liable or responsible for any loss or damage allegedly arising as a consequence of the use or application of any information or suggestions in this book.

Archway Publishing books may be ordered through booksellers or by contacting:

Archway Publishing
1663 Liberty Drive
Bloomington, IN 47403
www.archwaypublishing.com
1-(888)-242-5904

Because of the dynamic nature of the Internet, any web addresses or links contained in this book may have changed since publication and may no longer be valid. The views expressed in this work are solely those of the author and do not necessarily reflect the views of the publisher, and the publisher hereby disclaims any responsibility for them.

Cover photo courtesy and © Becton, Dickinson and Company.
Reprinted with permission.

ISBN: 978-1-4808-1090-7 (sc)
ISBN: 978-1-4808-1091-4 (e)

Library of Congress Control Number: 2014915454

Printed in the United States of America.

Archway Publishing rev. date: 10/1/2014

Dedication

To my wife, Terry—the love of my life—you are my constant encouragement, and to my sons, Paul and David, you are my inspiration.

And

To all nurses and paramedics, past and present, seasoned and novice, for all you do to help comfort and care for the sick, injured, and dying. You are a blessing to humanity.

"Accept the challenges, so that you may feel the exhilaration of victory." 　　　　　　—George S. Patton Jr

Contents

Introduction

The ability of any nurse or healthcare clinician to be successful when initiating a peripheral intravenous line (IV) is paramount to the successful outcome of the patient. The IV is virtually the patient's lifeline and is fundamental for the protection and preservation of life in a critical situation. It is the access by which fluids, medications, parenteral nutrition, and blood products are administered directly into the bloodstream when someone is truly ill. Without a properly placed IV, the patient quite often cannot be adequately treated and can deteriorate very rapidly. This is not to say that other, more invasive and costly accesses (peripherally inserted central catheter (PICC) line or a central venous catheter) cannot be inserted, but there are significant risks and increased costs associated with the placement of these lines. The standard peripheral IV is the most common and cost-effective technique for most patients, and if performed correctly, it enhances patient safety.

My experience and observation tell me this skill is lacking now more than ever, and that it needs to be properly learned by the novice nurse/clinician and even relearned by those who are experienced and providing direct patient care. As a bedside critical care nurse for nineteen years and an EMT/Paramedic for fifteen years, I have helped train many nurses in the art of proper IV technique.

Years ago in paramedic school, we used to stick an orange to get the *feel* of the procedure, and we even made one attempt initiating an IV on our classmate (however, this practice is not recommended today). We went to hospital laboratories to get the *feel* of puncturing human skin to find the vein and then draw blood. That was the extent of my training. I can tell you that the first time I went to stick a living, breathing human being; I was shaking like a leaf. As a new medical provider, I was in the land of the unknown, and it was pretty intimidating not having performed this procedure before.

Currently in nursing school, students spend a couple of hours at most reviewing the basics and then may practice starting an IV on an anatomical arm with bulging veins. That is usually the extent of their training. Some new nurses have even told me that their IV training was *minimal* at best, or say, *We just didn't talk about it a lot.* Also, the arm does not talk back or express all of the emotions a true patient can and quite often does.

The question that begs to be asked then is, *How can someone who is endowed with such an important responsibility to care for the sick and injured become proficient at initiating a patient's lifeline except for on-the-job training?* The assumption is always that experienced nurses will properly train new nurses on the necessary techniques for optimum success. My experience tells me differently, as I have witnessed a gradual decline over the years in the IV skill level of most nurses and other clinicians. Usually the specifics of the technique are most often unknown, missed, or forgotten and consequently never get passed on. The pure essence of successful IV initiation truly lies in the fine details of the procedure.

There are many very good medical surgical, emergency, and critical care nurses currently working who are lacking in expertise at starting IVs. This in no way implies that they are bad nurses. It only means that they need to refine their technique and not shy away from the difficult *sticks* (IVs). I am a firm believer that anyone can learn to be proficient at and comfortable with starting IVs. All you need is confidence in yourself, the determination to want to do it right the first time, and the knowledge of the fine details of initiating a peripheral IV. There is more to this than meets the eye.

Realistically speaking, the nurses, paramedics, or advanced clinicians who lack excellent IV skills are effectively handicapped in the care of their patients. They can only do a portion of the job they were hired to do, and because of their lack of this most essential skill, the patient may ultimately suffer if treatment is delayed. The problem is that this is an essential and critical part of the job for all bedside nurses and prehospital paramedics. All of the tender, loving care in the world cannot make up for the fact that critically ill patients or those going for routine surgery will be unable to receive their IV medications, fluids, or blood in a timely manner. Over the years, those who are now currently proficient in IV starts may transfer to other departments, go on for advanced degrees, or even retire from the healthcare profession. These factors will leave a crop of clinicians who are deficient, or at best, *average* in this most important skill.

Many nurses and clinicians practice the *Gee, I hope I get it,* multiple stick method of IV insertion. These persons are short on confidence. The Merriam-Webster online dictionary defines confidence as "a feeling or belief that you can do something well or succeed at something." I have witnessed many good nurses who are truly lacking in confidence when attempting an IV. As with any new technique, a certain skill level needs to be attained in order to become proficient. Practice makes perfect in starting IVs, and this process is no different (from the standpoint that practice makes perfect) than tying your shoes.

As we all learned how to tie our shoes, we fumbled around but kept at it until we worked out the bugs. We learned how to cross the shoelaces and make a loop. We learned how to pass one lace through the loop and pull tight to secure the knot. In essence, we first learned the coarse motor skill, and then by practice we learned the finesse of the procedure. The more we tied our shoes the better we became at doing it. This is what initiating an IV is like. You have to develop the skill or art of the procedure, and then develop your own finesse or refinement of that technique. The more you do, the better you will become if you practice the skills contained in this book. *Practice, practice, practice, coupled with perseverance, does make perfect.*

I am a huge proponent of the *one and done* philosophy, as I feel everyone should be. The goal of this book is to get you there and on track. One stick, one IV: less pain and discomfort for the patient, a higher level of confidence for the nurse or paramedic providing the best medical care, and a higher level of satisfaction and confidence by the patient that the care received is exceptional.

I feel passionate that by concentrating on the techniques included in this book, those nurses and clinicians responsible for initiating an intravenous line will achieve a higher level of confidence and discipline and learn that this is more of an art than a rote procedure. Every patient and situation is different; therefore, it takes poise and finesse to achieve success. Even if you are already good at initiating IVs, if you take away only one idea from this book, I feel you will become even better and stronger in your skill.

Initiating an IV on a patient is serious business. To be successful, you have to pay attention to the details. I can't stress this point enough. It's the small stuff that makes a big difference. Anyone can learn the major steps of starting an IV and run in the middle of the pack. I thought I was average, just like most, but it wasn't until I started to pay attention to the fine details that my success rate dramatically improved. So I encourage you to learn the small stuff and discipline yourself. Read the fine print, so to speak, and the big stuff will take care of itself.

Let me pause to say that, in spite of what you take away from these techniques, nothing takes the place of good, professional nursing judgment. These procedures should only act as a guide of what to look for and circumstances to consider when dealing with your patient. *You* are always responsible for knowing your anatomy, considering the circumstances involving your patient, familiarizing yourself with the equipment you are using, and knowing the medicines and fluids you will be administering.

As a professional, you are also obligated to abide by your state's Nurse Practice Act or paramedic standards and to familiarize yourself with the proper standards of care for peripheral intravenous lines. They are outlined by your respective medical organization's IV protocols and those found in the Infusion Nurses Society (INS) *Journal of Infusion Nursing: Infusion Nursing Standards of Practice.*

As you can see, starting a patient's peripheral IV carries with it a high level of responsibility. After all, you will be invading a patient's bloodstream, and you need to do it right the first time to limit and prevent any chance of risky complications.

Also, this is not an anatomy book, a physiology book, a physics book, or a chemistry book. Although the content included herein may touch upon some or all of these subjects, I make no claim as to the detail of why certain techniques work. All I know is that they *do* work. Discussion as to the *whys* and *hows* can be reserved for another day. Also, I do not know or have all the answers. I know I can learn as much from you as you will take away from this book. It only serves as an introduction or primer into the techniques needed to be a skilled IV clinician. Hopefully, this goal will be achieved, and you will gain your confidence.

Through the years, I have learned, adopted, analyzed, and gleaned some common-sense procedures that I trust, if applied correctly, will help enhance the success rate for initiating the standard peripheral IV. I am confident these techniques and little *tricks of the trade* will increase the morale and confidence of the nurse, paramedic, or clinician and the experience of the patient for the best possible outcomes. That's why I call this *The Art of the IV Start.* Let's therefore learn what this art is all about.

My Story

While living in rural New York State in the early 1980s, I became an EMT with our local volunteer fire department. Running calls as an EMT was fulfilling, but I always felt I could and should do more to help the sick and injured. I learned that there was a new phase of emergency medical services (EMS) where you could go on and become an advanced provider like the new paramedics in cities. Advanced life support (ALS) was now reaching rural communities, and I wanted to be a part of that.

I began my advanced training and obtained my IV certification on November 1, 1983, after practicing on an orange and then attempting to start an IV on one of my classmates. I was successful on my first attempt, but as with anything new, my technique was pretty clumsy. In any class, you learn the basics once and then move on to other class material. That was the extent of my IV training.

As my advanced training continued, I never had the opportunity to initiate another IV for a long time. I lived in a small community of about five thousand people and only ran EMS as a volunteer (as we all did back then), so the opportunity never truly presented itself. I truly feel, however, that with ALS being a new concept in the community, we were all afraid to take that first step to go above and beyond our basic EMT training.

Then on a warm Sunday morning, while lying in bed, I heard the tones go off and responded from home to an emergency call for a patient having chest pain. I knew I wouldn't get to the squad room in time to jump on the ambulance, so I took a back road, intercepted the ambulance, and followed them into the scene. Upon arriving at the scene, we found a middle-aged man sitting on the floor in the doorway of his upstairs bathroom, one leg in the bathroom and one leg in the hallway. He was ashen, diaphoretic, and complaining of severe, midsternal chest pain.

We put oxygen on him and figured we would load him up and transport to the hospital, as we always did. Suddenly, he cardiac arrested right in front of us without warning. My partner (who was also a cardiac technician) and I looked at each other and, at that moment, decided this was what we went to school for, so we should do what we were trained to do. Our other ambulance crew mates started CPR, and he and I worked to initiate our IV, airway, and defibrillation skills. That is when I experienced my first official prehospital IV.

We worked on this gentleman, giving him emergency medicine and other advanced life support skills and then transported him to the hospital, where they even gave him intra-cardiac epinephrine (remember, this is back in the early 1980s). Unfortunately, the outcome was less than desired, as the gentleman expired, but we took the first step and from that point on began to utilize our skills and perform ALS in the field. (Isn't it interesting how in health care we have to rely on other people getting sick so we can become good at what we do? If we are not good at our craft, we cannot help others.)

Fast forward to 1984; that is when my wife, Terry, and I moved to south central Pennsylvania. I began to run as a paramedic with the local ALS unit, and I felt I did pretty well at running calls and initiating IVs. Like everyone else, I got a few IVs and missed a few and felt I was pretty average. I didn't think it was a big deal to miss some of my IV sticks because, what the heck, everyone else did. Consequently, I felt comfortable with who I was and what I could do. I ran in the middle of the pack.

Then I hit the wall. I couldn't start an IV if you paid me. There I was supposed to be saving lives, yet I couldn't even hit the broad side of a barn. I missed one, then another, then another and felt I was just having a bad day or a bad couple of days. Let me tell you that after you get past four misses in a row, you begin to keep count. I kept missing and missing until I ran a streak of fifteen consecutive IV misses in a row.

While other nurses, paramedics, and even doctors were watching my technique, no one was able to determine what I was doing wrong. Everyone said my technique was good, but I just couldn't get the *stick*. I hit the bottom of my confidence level. *How can I save lives if I can't even initiate a patient's lifeline?* I thought. I was lost. My medical knowledge was sound, but my IV skill level was gone.

It was so bad that at our annual awards banquet, I received a gag award for my lack of proficiency. The chief of our ALS unit, my good friend, Mills, presented me with a book on acupuncture and said I was the area's first acupuncture specialist. Everyone knew of my trials and tribulations, but not one of the good nurses or paramedics I worked with ever lost confidence in me. Everyone was truly supportive and never gave up on me.

Then one day, I did it. I happened to be on duty one night, and we had a very sick patient in the ER. All of the other nurses couldn't get the IV; I was their last resort. Well again, everyone else missed, so what's one more if I should miss? To make a long story short, I got the IV. It was what we call a blind stick, where you can't visualize and, in this case, even palpate the vein. You are not really sure where the vein is, and you are only going by landmarks where you know the vein should be. I initiated the IV stick on my first attempt, and the patient didn't even feel the needle going in. What a relief. I then began to ponder, *What the heck just happened and why?*

From that point on, I became better at this fine art of IV initiation. Over time, I began to evaluate what techniques work and which ones don't. I've had the opportunity to evaluate, monitor, and refine my skills to a working set of fundamental techniques that I feel will help any new (or even older) practitioners become more successful. Included in this book are my words of wisdom that I think will help any practitioner become successful in the art of starting peripheral IVs.

As with any skill, there is a lot of finesse or fine tuning that goes into it, in addition to a lot of patience. The tips and techniques in the pages that follow are designed to help you, the practitioner, to think and evaluate, and then it is up to you to develop your own style. I have taught many nurses over the years, from novices to veterans, and have witnessed a significant increase of their IV skill sets. I believe if you adopt any or all of these tips, you will become proficient in this most-needed medical skill. Remember, practice makes perfect, and you should never shy away from an opportunity. Even if the stick is a difficult one, go for it. I know you can do it.

One critical bit of advice is to pay attention to the details. Your success depends on it.

Aseptic Technique

Proper aseptic technique is mandatory and is one of the most important steps you will ever take to initiate a safe and secure intravenous access. Everything else is secondary. Proper aseptic technique means cleansing and disinfecting the skin to remove harmful microorganisms and prevent infection prior to penetrating the skin. I don't care how good you become at starting IVs; it is all meaningless if you cannot disinfect the site properly to prevent infection. Remember, your patient's health is at risk. Usually patients are already in a compromised state (they are ill and have low or stressed immune systems), and they do not need more insult to injury by getting an infection from someone with poor aseptic technique. *Excellent asepsis is mandatory, period.*

First, I wash or disinfect my hands before approaching my patient. This is just good practice. I will then always look at my possible sites first and find my vein initially without using gloves, if I can, unless bodily fluids are present or the patient has a transmissible disease. (Medics in the field must always use gloves before they approach any of their patients). Once you know where you want to go, you then must always adhere to *universal precautions* by putting on a pair of gloves. This is a must and can't be stressed enough. This is the initiation of your proper aseptic technique. Usually non-latex gloves would be preferred in case the patient has a latex allergy.

Most IV start kits come with gloves already included, and they are okay to use, but I find these usually do not fit me properly. I prefer very tight-fitting gloves to enhance better needle/catheter control and so I can feel the vein when I palpate. (Yes, if you really pay attention, you can most often feel the vein with gloves on.) I don't like having slack or space at the fingertip. (I normally wear medium-sized gloves for general tasks but prefer to use small gloves when initiating IVs.) If you wear gloves that have slack at the fingertips, it will create a hindrance to feeling the vein properly and promotes clumsy technique. Be sure your gloves are nice and tight.

To properly prepare the skin, you need to take the antiseptic applicator (usually Chlorhexidine) contained in most standard IV start packs, and scrub the site. I have witnessed many nurses who only wet the skin with antiseptic by lightly rubbing it over the site, but they do no actual scrubbing of the site. You need to be somewhat abrasive, rubbing off at least several layers of dead skin to remove a majority of the normal skin flora and transient contaminating bacteria.

Be cautious with patients who have sensitive skin, however, because being overly aggressive with older or fragile patients, or those that are on anticoagulant therapy, can cause a hematoma or bruising under the skin. You need to avoid this at all cost. When treating these patients, you want to be gently abrasive but not overly aggressive. Light friction is the key. (One advantage I have found to properly scrubbing the site is that rubbing over the vein will often times cause it to pop up more, if it was not evident at first.) Once you scrub the site for at least ten-to-fifteen seconds, allow the antiseptic to dry.

Bacteria die off at an exponential rate over time. This is why you need to allow the antiseptic time to dry. If you perform your IV stick too soon while the antiseptic is still wet, you can still introduce some microorganisms into the blood stream and also cause an increased stinging discomfort to the patient by introducing the antiseptic into the puncture site. (Yes, I know that the needle will also sting the site.) Once the skin is properly prepared, you are now ready to stick the site. Good asepsis requires that you never re-palpate or touch a site that has already been disinfected.

Knowing Your Equipment—
Over the Needle Catheters

IV catheters come in sizes from 14 gauges to 24 gauges, and the numbers have an inverse proportion to their bore size. The higher the number the smaller the size or bore. As paramedics, our standard prehospital size to use was an 18 gauge. Trauma sizes were typically 16 gauges for the administration of large volumes of fluids, but keep in mind that many prehospital mobile intensive care units (MICUs) may not carry pumps and need to rely on IV pressure infusers. Many hospitals use smaller gauges as their normal starting size (usually 20 or 22 gauge catheters), as conditions are more controlled, and these sizes are more comfortable and less painful for patients. Plus, they can still accept large volumes of fluid when placed on an IV pump.

What I have found is that you become what you get used to. If you are used to starting 18s, then you get good at inserting that size. If you get used to inserting 22s, again, that becomes your comfort level. You always need to adhere to your hospital's protocol or doctor's order when initiating an IV, and you need to become proficient at that level.

As with any circumstance, however, there is usually some leeway in which to choose a different sized catheter. Every patient is different. Some have bulging veins that are very elastic and can tolerate a larger bore, whereas diabetic patients usually have very fragile, fine, *spider*-type veins. Also, don't get too comfortable or *cocky* when you see a bulging vein, as sometimes they are more difficult to get because of their elasticity. I have had first-hand experience at this and have blown many big veins I thought would be easy to get. If you are too overconfident, then that is the time you will usually miss the stick. The best advice I can offer is this: in every

IV attempt, be humble; always keep your guard up, and approach every IV with a very high degree of discipline.

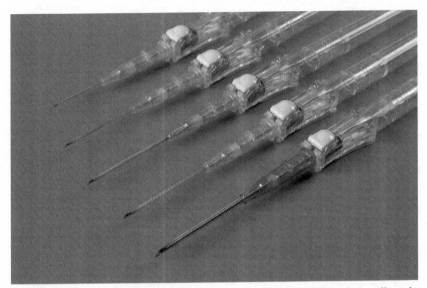

Catheter sizes: This image shows the most common sizes of IV over the needle catheter devices (16 gauge-24 gauge). Note the various lengths of catheters depending on size and how the catheter sits behind the bevel of the needle. (Image of BD Insyte™ Autoguard™ IV catheters Courtesy and © Becton, Dickinson and Company. Reprinted with permission)

Every IV attempt must be approached with the same caution, formality, and discipline as the next. You will, however, have to use your best professional judgment when selecting the size catheter you want to use. Keep in mind that you need to make a rational estimate to always assure that the catheter is smaller than the lumen of the vein so that blood flow is always maintained around the inserted catheter.

I have seen both nurses and medics pound their chest about using larger than needed gauges inappropriately. One instance in particular was when a paramedic was *strutting his stuff* about getting a 16 gauge in a patient's hand. That is inappropriate. To begin with, the patient was not that critical, and the same treatment could have been achieved with a smaller gauge catheter. What's the point of using that size in that situation? He thought he was a big deal, and the only reason he gave for using such a large needle was that the patient's veins were big and that he could.

The point I am trying to make is that you need to get comfortable with what your hospital or medic unit protocol dictates, but that doesn't mean you can't think outside the box in certain situations; just be appropriate about it. Some procedures require larger bores because IV contrast is infused under pressure (IV contrast for CAT scan in particular). Conversely, if you have a patient with many tiny veins and you think you can only get a 24 gauge, then get the IV with a 24 gauge.

Always remember, the peripheral IV is the patient's lifeline—*period*. Don't ever allow someone make you feel inferior about using a smaller gauge. The point is, you are the one who got the IV, and he/she didn't. In critical, life-threatening situations, my rule of thumb is to anticipate going big, but get what you can get. If you get a smaller gauge IV first, then you can worry about a larger bore (if needed) when you have more time to look.

In removing the needle from the protective enclosure, do so cautiously because abruptly pulling the cap off can cause the plastic catheter to slide up or sometimes off the needle. Also, if you do this abruptly (as I see some do), think of how this is perceived by the patient. You pick up the over the needle catheter, hastily pull off the protective cap, and tell the patient they will *feel a stick*. At that point, they probably feel that you are now ready to *stab* them because they will see your hasty action as being overly aggressive. Perception is everything, and you always need to exude a calm confidence about what you do. One of the most important things to achieve success is to put your patient at ease.

To properly remove the protective cap, you need to be in control and gently loosen it, being careful not to dislodge the plastic over-the-needle catheter from around the needle. Now that you are holding the needle/catheter combination, you need to only turn the catheter a quarter turn or less to loosen it on the needle. Never slide the catheter up and down over the needle because the bevel end is very sharp and could result in internal damage of the catheter causing shear, which could produce micro-emboli. This is bad practice.

Needle/bevel/catheter design:

Knowing the design and relationship of the plastic catheter to the IV needle is another important piece of information for knowing how to achieve success. *This may very well be the most significant fact needed to becoming truly proficient.* Most practitioners usually pay no attention to this factor or are uninformed about it, but *this* design is *that* significant. It may seem common to an experienced clinician, but to the novice nurse or paramedic, it is not on their list of priorities.

If you look at the bevel end of the needle, you will see that the plastic catheter sits at the end of or behind the bevel, roughly about one to two millimeters behind the sharp tip of the needle. With the smaller bore (i.e., 24 gauge), the catheter is only a little over one millimeter behind the bevel, whereas with the larger bore (i.e., 16 gauge), the catheter is a little over two millimeters behind the bevel. (Refer to "Catheter sizes" image). As you can see, it is not flush with the needle tip, as many think. Knowing this bit of information will positively impact your success rate in more ways than you can imagine. Now tuck this bit of information away, and we will discuss why it is so important in a subsequent chapter. This is all you need to know for now.

Secure the catheter:

If you look at the design of the IV needle/catheter combination, many have recessed finger grips, while others may have *wings* with which to hold the needle device. Once you loosen the catheter by a quarter turn, you need to assure it is stabilized or secure so that it does not slide or *float up and down on the needle after you puncture the skin.*

Once the needle punctures the skin, the skin will create resistance and provide drag on the plastic catheter. If you are not securing the loosened catheter to the needle in some way and you miss the vein and have to *fish* around for it, as you pull the needle in and out trying to find the vein, the catheter will lag behind or be delayed while only the needle will be moving. This can cause internal problems that can blow the vein. The catheter should always stay behind the bevel of the needle once the puncture is made and you are under the skin.

I have seen some clinicians hold the needle device with their thumb and index finger at the recessed finger grips, not securing the catheter at all. Others hold the needle device with three fingers by using the thumb and middle finger of their dominant hand to hold the recessed finger grips while their index finger holds the catheter secure at the twelve o'clock (or top) position. This places the hand and wrist at an unnatural angle, thus making it more difficult and uncomfortable for the nurse/clinician to access the vein. Comfort is mandatory to being successful at the bedside.

I suggest that the more natural and comfortable way to do this is to always hold the needle and catheter so that the index finger of your dominant hand secures the catheter hub at the two o'clock position for right hand-dominant and at the ten o'clock spot for left hand-dominant clinicians. To do this, half of your index finger will be on the plastic needle holder distal to the finger recess area, while the other half of your finger will be securing the hub of the catheter. (See image "Secure the catheter"). Putting your index finger at the two o'clock point positions the wrist at a more natural (I estimate roughly thirty-to-forty-five degree angle) and increases the comfort of the clinician, allowing for easier access.

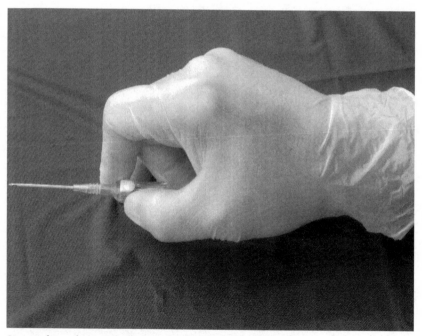

Secure the catheter: This image shows the suggested method of securing the catheter before and during the IV attempt and shows how the index finger is half on the catheter hub and half on the needle holder at the two o'clock spot. This places the hand and wrist at a more comfortable angle and position to allow easier access to the vein. (BD Insyte™ Autoguard™ IV catheter shown courtesy of Becton, Dickinson and Company)

When you hold the catheter this way as you move the needle in and out, you can be sure the catheter always remains stationary. It will not float along the needle, thus causing catheter shear and a greater chance of blowing the vein. This is a fundamental principle you have to adapt to and condition yourself for to achieve greater success. Implementation of this procedure will dramatically improve your success rate for initial IV sticks.

Tourniquet above the Elbow

Two big problems I have seen are that many nurses put their tourniquet too low on the arm (below the elbow), and they put their tourniquet on too loosely. Now when I say it's too loose, that is a relative statement. They usually think it's on tight enough, but quite often, it is not tight enough to fully engorge the veins with blood. I believe most clinicians are afraid to put the tourniquet on as tight as is needed for fear of hurting the patient.

For optimum success, always place a *tight* tourniquet *above* the elbow, and place it tight enough to compress the veins. I always put my tourniquet on tighter than most; this allows the veins to fill better. Some patients will say, "Boy, that's tight!" but I always inform them before applying my tourniquet. You need to be sure, however, not to put it on so tight that you restrict blood flow in the arteries, and you also need to maintain some minor blood flow in the veins. It is the finesse of the procedure that you have to develop. It is a professional judgment call. Due to the fact that my tourniquet is tighter than most, I will quite often wrap it around the sleeve of the patient's hospital gown to avoid cutting into or pinching the patient's skin.

Placing the tourniquet above the elbow allows you to see all of the landmarks in the hand and forearm and not restrict yourself from viewing what might be a good vein. If you place it at mid-forearm, like I see many nurses do, you will miss detecting some very nice veins higher up. When you are initially looking, why would you want to hinder yourself from seeing everything you need to see? You need to give yourself a wide open field. Obviously, if the patient has a PICC line in the same arm and you need another access (as quite often happens in critical care), place the tourniquet below the PICC if the other arm is unavailable.

What used to be the rule seems now to have become the exception to the rule. Thirty years ago, it was standard to look at the hands first and initiate your IV there, if at all possible. Today I find that most nurses, for some reason, stay away from the hand. I don't know why. Some of the best veins you will ever find are in the hand, and for most general patients this is a perfectly fine and acceptable access site.

The rule of thumb you always want to follow is to *start low (distal) and work high (proximal)*. This practice has been around for years, but for some unknown reason, many novice nurses fail to abide by this rule. I have witnessed countless nurses going for an IV in the forearm initially, instead of first looking in the hand. For most large bore, high volume IVs you may have to start higher; however, I estimate at least two-thirds or more of all common IVs can be started in the hand.

It is so important to start low on the arm because if you miss low and have to go higher, you reduce the chance of infiltration. We once received a critical patient in our ICU who needed emergent IV access, and we didn't have a surgeon on staff (at 2:00 a.m.) to put in a central line. Other nurses tried and were unsuccessful in initiating the IV. They asked me to initiate one, but I was in an isolation room with my own patient and had to finish a procedure first before I could try.

One of our very good newer nurses wanted to try because she loved a challenge. She attempted to access a vein high up near the antecubital but also missed. The patient was filled with edema, and by the time I looked, the patient's arm was covered with multiple small dressings. Even after removing these, I couldn't see any of the landmarks. I finally got an IV in the patient's thumb, but when we ran the fluid in, we infiltrated in the upper arm where the previous nurse had stuck. Finally, we called in a surgeon to put in a central line on this patient.

The point is, if you stick high first and miss, you are putting your patient at risk for an infiltrate if you then get an IV lower in the hand or arm. Always start low and work high.

Landmarks—Know Your Anatomy

What seems to be common practice for a lot of nurses/clinicians today is to put the tourniquet on and look for any vein anywhere to pop up. If they don't see something obvious, they then start poking around for something visible or a spongy vein under the skin, but quite often, they are just *shot-gunning* their approach. Many clinicians have no system for finding a vein. This is often because they truly feel they are looking for a vein but aren't really sure where to look. You can do better.

Knowing the location or general vicinity of the most prominent veins in the hands and forearms is crucial to success. It is not important to know the names of the respective veins (although for your knowledge, that would be a plus), but if you know *where* to look, you give yourself a greater chance of finding a vein that no one else sees, especially those veins that are deep under the skin or can't be seen due to excessive edema or even thick skin. Knowing your anatomy is extremely important to good IV success. I can't stress this point enough.

As I said earlier, the hand veins are some of the best veins you will ever see. The skin there is thinner in most patients, and you can see the veins more readily. I have heard some nurses say that they stay away from the hand because an IV there is more painful to the patient, or that it causes interference when a patient eats or bathes. The point is that if a patient needs a lifeline and a nurse has mediocre or average skills, do you really want to struggle with the deeper veins of the forearm and risk multiple sticks, or do you want to stick the patient once and be done with it? Multiple IV sticks not only cause the patient unnecessary pain, but more importantly, they open the patient up to increased risk of infection. *I opt for one and done.* Therefore, always look for an IV in the hand first. First rule of order is to always start low and work high.

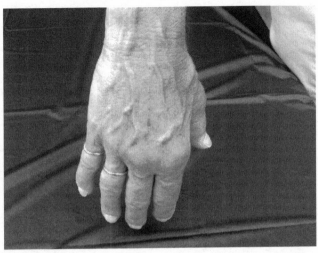

Hand veins: Note the various choice options of hand veins. Notice the bifurcated veins. These are optimum veins to access when initiating an IV.

As you move proximally up the arm, the cephalic vein presents nicely as it passes the lateral aspect (anatomic position) of the wrist. This is a beautiful vein to go for, but I reserve it as a last resort. Some educators say to stay away from this vein because of the nerves in the wrist; however, when you go for it you should not be sticking in the wrist but just above it. Obviously, you do not want to stick an IV at a joint or bend point where the catheter can kink, but in a critical emergency, if you have to, you have to. You can always stabilize the joint after the fact. As the cephalic travels up the lateral aspect of the arm, it begins to branch off and presents itself with other excellent options.

Usually there are two nice, deep veins in the anterior aspect of the forearm—one of them being the median antebrachial vein. These veins are a little deeper than most, but they are also more stable than most because they are supported by muscle on each side and have less tendency to roll.

The basilic vein travels up the posterior medial aspect of the forearm and also presents nicely with several branches to cannulate. To access the basilic vein, you need to bend the patient's arm at the elbow upward and outward.

Remember, it is very important that all IV sticks are placed with the catheter tip pointing toward the heart along with the normal flow of blood.

A right hand-dominant person starting an IV on the basilic vein of the patient's right arm must always remember this. The same is true on the left side if you are left hand-dominant and are starting an IV on the patient's left arm. To access properly, you must bend the patient's arm outward, or you must readjust your stance appropriately. A simple trick to see and access this vein better is to reposition the patient on his/her side with the arm up. (Who says the patient has to just be sitting upright or lying flat in bed?)

Then there are the antecubital veins. These are large veins and are nice for running high volume fluids; they are also the best veins for pushing the emergency medicine, Adenosine. Adenosine is a medicine that has such a short half-life that it is best to deliver this into the closest peripheral vein to the heart. I reserve the antecubital veins as a last resort because the bend at the elbow kinks the catheter. However, in an emergency, or if you can't find anything else, you have to go for it to save the patient's life.

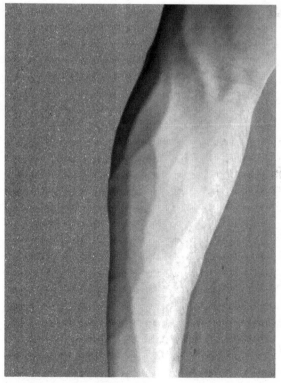

Forearm veins: The forearm also presents with various good options to access. Notice the bifurcated veins. These are more stable than straight veins.

Once your tourniquet is applied (above the elbow), and you have an idea which vein you are going to access, you need to get the vein to rise up. It needs to engorge with blood so you can see it or palpate it. Engorgement of blood does not necessarily get the vein to appear every time, however. You have to get the vein to dilate, as it is made of smooth muscle. Do not be afraid to *flick* the vein with your finger or *pat* the vein with the fingers of your hand to get it to come up. As I tell my students, *you have to "whack it, pat it, flick it, or smack it."*

Now don't get alarmed. Some of you may find the above statement to be *strong language* and find it offensive. I am not advocating harming the patient in any way, but I am trying to make a point.

Obviously, you are never going to abuse the patient, and you have to be careful if patients are on blood thinners, as you can cause hemorrhaging under the skin if you are too aggressive. So before you proceed, you need to inform your patient of what you are going to do. Do not be afraid to work the vein. Remember, you want to do the IV right the first time; in order to do this, it is best to see your target.

I know the *whack it, pat it, flick it, or smack it* technique is old school, but I can tell you from my thirty years of experience, it does work and should be used to get the vein to rise and dilate. I cannot tell you the mechanism involved causing this to happen, but it is a very real phenomenon. It is almost like the vein spasms in reverse and causes itself to dilate. Again, you need to keep your patient informed about what you are doing. (Remember also, if you have a potential vein you want to go for, often times scrubbing the site during aseptic technique causes it to become more pronounced and give a better presentation).

Finding the Difficult Vein

If the vein is stubborn and does not want to come up, try some of these tricks:

Let gravity work for you. After applying your tourniquet, try hanging the patient's arm over the side of the bed or gurney (stretcher), and let gravity fill the vein. While doing this, continue to flick the vein to help it engorge with blood.

Apply a warm compress. Sometimes this is just enough to see the vein and get it to rise. Warmth will take a constricted vein and dilate it so that it is more accessible.

Obviously, all of this is more difficult if the patient is hypotensive or volume depleted. This is where your skill will really be tested. The veins in hypotensive patients are hard to find, but if you know your landmarks, you will have an edge over the clinician who is just looking for anything but does not truly know where to look. You do not want to be average; you want to be great at what you do. Believe me when I say, your patient will be grateful that you are competent at what you do.

Press out the fluid. When a patient has significant edema, you can do all of the looking you want, and you are not going to see your common landmarks. Fluid within the skin and under the skin increases its thickness and hides the veins. This is where knowing your landmarks becomes important. If you know where to look, take the thumbs of both your hands and press firmly over the site where you suspect (or know) the vein to be. Hold pressure for ten, fifteen, or twenty seconds; then look to see if you can see the blue streak of the vein. Do this several times if needed. If you can't see the vein you are looking for, don't give up. Go to another landmark location and repeat the process.

The hand is probably the easiest area on which to perform this process because the veins are more prominent here, but you can be equally successful anywhere on the forearm. Once the fluid is displaced, *whack it, pat it, flick it, and smack it* to get the vein to pop up. This simple technique will greatly enhance your chances of finding a vein to cannulate.

Moisten the site. What happens when a patient has dry skin? Quite often you can look for a vein and vaguely see it. You know it's there, you think you see it, but it's not very apparent. One little trick to try to enhance the visibility of the vein is to take a damp paper towel or washcloth, or even use the Chlorhexidine antiseptic applicator, and wipe over the site you are observing. Simple moistening of the skin greatly enhances the visibility of the veins underneath; it's a simple technique, yet very effective. Keep in mind that if you use the Chlorhexidine applicator to moisten the skin, you are not aseptically scrubbing the site. You are simply just moistening the skin to see the vein better. After you decide which vein you want to stick, you still need to perform your proper aseptic procedure.

Mark the site. Most novice clinicians usually assume that when starting an IV, they can always see the vein. Visualization of the vein provides a comfortable feeling for most, but it is not always realistic. In a perfect world this would be the case, but in reality, some veins cannot be seen— only felt. Then there are times when you cannot even feel the vein. (You need to know where your landmarks are.) Some patients have deep veins, while others have thick skin that hinders seeing the blue streak of the vein. Usually, however, you can palpate the sponginess of the vein under the skin with a gentle, light pressure with your fingertip. Once you find the vein, you can usually trace it and find how it tracks under the skin.

When there's a vein that can be felt but not seen, I have often witnessed nurses and medics go for the *blind stick* by disinfecting the site and then retouching the vein just before they stick because they can't visualize it. They do this because they want to make sure they are sticking in the right spot. First off, this is very poor aseptic technique. Secondly, they are usually off-mark when attempting the IV because, even though they fish around for it, they fail to compensate for vein shift when applying proper traction. Presented with these circumstances, many clinicians will often miss the vein. In these cases you have to come up with another technique to improve your chances of hitting the vein on the first stick. When presented with this *blind stick* scenario, you need to *mark the site.*

Marking the site will greatly increase your success rate. You do not just mark the vein where it sits, however. To improve your chances, you have to apply mild-to-moderate traction on the vein, all the while watching how the vein shifts. Your traction should be with your nondominant hand and should be in a downward and away motion. I want to stress that this traction is *mild* or *moderate* because you only want to see how the vein shifts before you place your mark. The vein always shifts in the direction of the traction.

Once you see the shift, palpate the vein again while holding traction, and mark the vein by gently pressing in with your fingernail and leaving an indentation on the skin. Your mark can be either horizontal across the vein or vertical along the vein tract. (I prefer a horizontal mark.) This gives you a frame of reference and vein access should be easier.

Next, after you scrub and disinfect the site (using good aseptic technique), you will see your *mark* and know you are on the vein, or at the very least, in the general vicinity when you go to stick. This minimizes fishing around and feeling lost as to where the vein might be. By marking the site, you have increased your chances of a *one and done* many times over. This also helps to prevent re-touching the already clean aseptic site before you stick for the vein. (I recommend that you perfect this technique, as tattooing and arm-sleeve body art are now mainstream, and quite often you cannot properly visualize typical vein presentation in these patients.) You will have to feel for the vein.

Remember, every step you take in preparation improves your chances and gives you the advantage for doing it right the first time, thus saving the patient needless pain and multiple sticks. One way to enhance the particular skill of marking your site is to perform this on veins you can see. I recommend making a mark directly on a visible vein, then pull moderate traction and re-mark the vein. This will allow you to get a stronger sense of how the vein shifts with traction, and you will develop a better perspective as your experience grows. Good luck.

Lastly, after you find the vein you want, remove your tourniquet. Yes, that's what I said, remove the tourniquet. I have found that many times during the looking process, if an inordinate amount of time is taken, then too much pressure can build up in the vein. Assuredly, I am not suggesting that you hurry. You only want to do that if an emergent crisis presents itself, and you have no IV access.

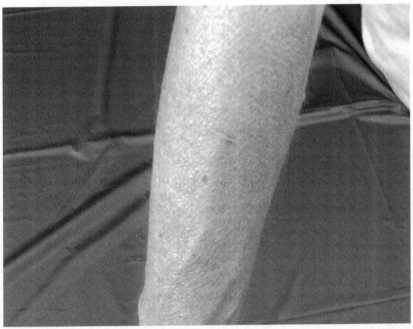

Mark the site: When a vein can be felt under the skin but cannot be seen, it is ideal to *mark* the vein before you aseptically cleanse the site. Notice the *fingernail* mark where the vein exists under the skin after mild to moderate traction was applied.

I am, however, suggesting that you take your time to look, and be sure you go for the best vein you feel comfortable with. If you have the time and take a long time to look, when you go to stick, sometimes the vein will blow because it has overly engorged and has built up too much back pressure. By releasing the tourniquet for fifteen-to-twenty seconds, the vein can relax its dilation/spasm, and the pressure inside re-equilibrates. Be sure to reapply the tourniquet again to get your vein back.

I have also found sometimes that when nurses take too long to find a vein, the reverse can happen, and the vein cannot maintain its dilation or spasm and needs to relax. Remember, veins have a thin layer of smooth muscle, and normal muscles cannot maintain spasm indefinitely. Once they reach a certain *point of no return*, they have to relax. Ironically, this is quite often the point when the nurse goes to stick the vein, and the vein then disappears. You can alleviate most of this flaw by releasing the tourniquet for a short time before re-applying and then prepping the site.

Go for the Bifurcate

You should always have several ideas of where you want to go with an IV. What do you do, however, when you are looking for your landmarks and you see this (Illustration 1): straight veins and bifurcated veins (veins that have a Y-site)? Which one do you want to go for?

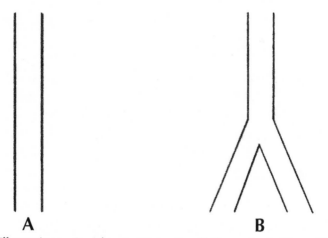

A   **B**

Illustration 1—Straight vein (Figure A) and bifurcated vein (Figure B).

Hint: There is no wrong answer.

Most nurses would say that Figure A is best because it is a straight shot into the vein and offers fewer potential problems. A few would say that Figure B is best because you have three potential areas to stick instead of one. (You can possibly stick both arms of the Y-site, or go directly for the long leg.) Again, both answers may be right, but there is a better option. (See Illustration 2)

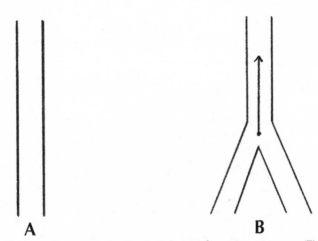

Illustration 2—Insert directly into the bifurcate for optimum success (Figure B).

Most nurses choose to go for the straight vein because it is a direct shot into the vein. This is not a bad option and is a correct response, but straight veins have a greater tendency to roll right or left, even if you are applying good traction. It takes a lot to properly anchor a straight vein. (We will talk about proper vein traction in a subsequent chapter.)

When presented with both options, *choose the bifurcated vein*, and go directly into the Y-site at the bifurcate (See Illustration 2, Figure B). The better choice is the bifurcated vein because it is more stable. The two shorter arms of this type vein serve to support and create a better anchor point, thus providing more stability and prevent rolling. Consider also that the higher up you go on the bifurcated vein you increase the chance for rolling, just like the straight vein. This is why you go directly into the bifurcate, as it is more securely anchored. Providing proper traction and anchoring of the vein is still imperative, however, as stabilization means everything toward achieving success.

Valves:

Now here's another dilemma. How do you select a vein when you have a patient with very noticeable valves? What if the valves are very close together? What approach will you use? The rule of thumb is to stay away from these, if at all possible, and look for another site. However, sometimes this is unavoidable. We do not live in a perfect world, and you may not have another option. Also, what about a patient in whom you can't see the valves at all? How do you know where they are? The problem is that you don't know.

So let's break this down. When you can see the valves, one approach would be to go beneath the valve (distally) far enough away where you hope the catheter tip will not rest up against it after the catheter is advanced. If the catheter tip is up against the valve, this would occlude a free flowing IV, and these are what we call *positional* IVs.

You may have to pull back on the catheter and tape it into place to prevent it from being *positional*. I know that the optimum IV is one in which the catheter is fully advanced (to the hilt), but you can still securely tape the IV in place after pulling the catheter back slightly to maintain the IV successfully. You may feel uneasy with these steps, but remember, you are still going to check on these frequently, as a good clinician always does. As long as you can draw blood back, these are perfectly good IVs. I have initiated many of these over the years with equal success.

Always apply a tourniquet first, and use a small, three milliliter syringe if you are trying to assess the patency of your IV and get a blood return. Remember, the tourniquet engorges the vein; however, use of a large syringe can cause too much suction that can collapse the vein and not yield any blood return. The smaller syringe provides less suction and less chance of collapsing the vein. As long as you can draw blood back (on your newly established IV), your IV is patent.

A second approach is to try to access above the valve (proximally) and bypass it. Again, you hope you have a long enough straight portion of the vein where you can achieve free flow without hindrance. I say go for it, and get your stick.

What about the veins where you can't see valves at all? It's not that you don't consider them. You know they are present, but the big issue is where they are located. One trick to try after applying your tourniquet is to occlude the vein distally with the thumb of one hand, and squeeze along the vein (in the direction of blood flow) with the other hand to collapse it and push the blood forward. By doing this, you are pushing the blood from that section of vein up to and past the next valve. The vein portion above the next valve will remain engorged, while the section you squeezed will become flat. Now you know where the valve is located and can avoid it. Once you release the distal pressure on the vein, you will see the collapsed vein section refill. Keep in mind, it fills quickly. This is a good way to find a valve. However, it is really only beneficial for a person who has large, noticeable veins to begin with. This does not work well for persons with thin, fragile veins.

Truthfully, during my whole career, I have never worried about valves. I truly think an inordinate amount of emphasis is placed on vein valves, especially when you need an IV immediately. It is not to say that they are not important to consider, but they are really not of great concern to me. I do not lose any sleep over them, but I will avoid them when I see them.

When you have patients with very small, thin veins, you are rarely ever going to know where the valves are. In this case, my best advice about valves is, *Forget about it*. It's not that it wasn't in the back of your mind, but you get what you can get, and don't worry about the valves. The most important thing here is, when you get flashback and try to advance the catheter, if you begin to meet resistance, don't force it. You may actually have stuck where a valve is and will have to *float the catheter* in. We will discuss more about floating the catheter in a subsequent chapter. It is a special technique that will greatly increase your success.

Your Comfort Is More Important than Your Patient's

I want to now talk about the comfort factor. One of the biggest problems I see when nurses try to start an IV is that many times they are out of position and are not at ease with what they are doing. Unknowingly, they are creating self-inflicted difficulty. It's the little things that count.

One rule I have always followed is, *Your comfort is more important than your patient's.* I know this goes against all nursing philosophy, but it is true when initiating an IV. Think about this. When surgeons put in a central line or perform a surgical procedure, they position the patient in the optimum way to achieve a successful outcome, and they position themselves for optimum comfort and control. Why shouldn't you? Proper positioning of the patient and/or patient's arm is just as vital to you when starting a peripheral IV, and you should take all necessary steps to control your environment for your optimum comfort. Remember, this is an invasive procedure and needs to be done right—the first time.

I see nurses sitting down, bending over too much, not moving a night stand out of the way, or not putting a side rail down, etc. Think about it; can you ever achieve success if *you* are not relaxed or comfortable?

I admit that I am not a fan of sitting in a chair when starting an IV. I see nurses doing this all the time. By sitting in a chair, you limit or lose your freedom of movement. A chair is too confining. It prevents you from stepping around as you look at the arm. It prevents you from bending and twisting the arm to see all that you should see. Just think about it. When you get a blood draw for personal lab work, do the phlebotomists sit in a chair? No. They are always standing because it gives them better access, and it helps enhance their skill.

Those who sit to start an IV usually hang the patient's arm way out over the side of the bed, then position a chair at the bedside and proceed to look for a vein. This is an unstable situation. First of all, by hanging the arm out over the side of the bed, there is no stability. Often, I see that the patient is too close to the edge of the bed, and the patient's arm is just sticking out. The arm is free to move or *flop around*, if you will. Then when you stick the skin, if the patient suddenly jerks his/her arm away, you automatically lose control.

Control is everything. The patient's arm should be resting on something. Whether it is resting on the bed, your knee, a table, or other stationary device, the arm must be stabilized and secure to achieve success. Again, think of a phlebotomist drawing your blood. Your arm is always stable.

I am a stander; I do not sit in a chair. Chair sitting is too confining and limiting because you significantly restrict your movement and cannot attain your comfort level. Freedom of movement for the IV initiator is imperative. In the hospital or clinic setting you have every opportunity to control your environment. Why not take it?

Paramedics who find themselves in awkward and compromising positions may have to squat, kneel, or even lay on their stomachs to gain IV access. Obviously, those in the prehospital arena are in an uncontrolled environment and need to adapt themselves to the situation. This is where finesse comes in. Been there, done that.

Quite often, the paramedic starts his/her IV in the back of the ambulance, sitting on the bench seat. That's right; they are in a sitting position, but in this case, the ambulance bench seat is close to the gurney, is usually at the same height as the patient, and the patient's arm can most often be stabilized properly.

When you set yourself up, be sure that everything surrounding you is for your benefit. Move items out of your way. Open up your field. Try standing at the bedside, but raise the bed to your comfort level. Don't bend over (save your back). Put your side rails down. Always position the patient in such a way as to afford you the best access and stability of his/her arm. You can try putting their arm up on a pillow or rolling your patient slightly on their side. If you need to raise or lower the patient's arm, do it. How about asking your patient to slide over a little in bed so the arm is resting on the bed? This provides more stability to the arm. All of these *little things* help you optimize and control your circumstance and put you in a more advantageous position. This may sound obvious and maybe even frivolous to some clinicians, but in my experience, it is often overlooked or not practiced. Always set yourself up for success.

The important thing to remember is to consistently keep your patient informed as to what you are doing and why you need to do it. Most often, they are scared and know that starting an IV is going to hurt. Always show confidence. Never let them see you sweat. A calm patient, a controlled environment, and a relaxed stance by the IV initiator will always make your life and your IV stick easier. If you do it right the first time, they will be eternally grateful.

Now because we talked about standing as the optimum position to initiate an IV, at the bedside, that doesn't mean unique circumstances will not present themselves. If your patient is already sitting in a chair, you will have to improvise. You may then have to sit in a chair yourself, or crouch down, or kneel on one knee, but again, these are unique situations. There are always exceptions to the rule.

Always be open-minded and maintain your flexibility, but do things to enhance your freedom of movement. (For example, move the bed out of the way, turn the patient's chair forty-five or ninety degrees to better access the arm, or lay the patient's arm on the bedside table, or kneel on one knee, and stabilize the patient's arm on your other knee.) Paramedics always find a way to improvise. That is what they are trained to do.

Once you find the vein you want (remember to release the tourniquet to re-establish venous flow and relieve pressure in the vein), place an absorbent pad or towel under your proposed puncture point. This will help keep your bed linens from becoming soiled with blood in the event your catheter leaks when withdrawing the needle. Open your IV start pack, and rip your tape into three equal strips about four inches long so that they are readily available. I will explain how to tape your IV securely in a later chapter.

Most hospital IVs are attached to extension tubing (either single access or y-site), primed with sterile saline. You need to set this up, and be sure you have a needleless cap on the end. You are now ready to go for it. Everything you need to secure the site is available; and the only thing needed now is the most important thing—getting the stick. We are now ready to access the vein.

Traction and Stabilization Are Everything

Traction, traction, traction! This is the essence of what we do. Once you know your landmark or the vein you are going to stick, traction on the vein and stabilization of the stick will help assure greater success. Now that you know how to hold the catheter (refer to image: *Secure the Catheter*), it is imperative to apply *proper* traction to the vein. I stress the word proper because my experience has shown that most clinicians do not know how to apply the *very firm* traction needed for true vein stabilization.

Traction is the act of *drawing or pulling*. Traction on the vein is the purposeful drawing down or pulling down of the skin and underlying tissue to cause the vein to tighten, lengthen, and reduce *roll*. Notice that I used the term, *drawing down*. This is important. *You always want to draw the skin and vein in the distal direction.* You *do not* want to draw upward or proximally.

I have witnessed various ways nurses draw traction. Some will draw down. Others will use their index finger and thumb to stretch the skin in opposite directions to attempt stabilization. Others will just use their thumb to draw the vein upward or proximal, thinking this is good stabilization. So let's break down and analyze each of these forms of traction.

Stabilize the vein:

First, one of my cardinal rules is never to place any finger above the stick point. This is not only bad form, but it really does not stabilize the vein at all. You run the risk of going for the vein and *slipping*, if you will, or going through the skin and giving yourself a dirty needle stick because your focus will be on finding the vein and not thinking about where your fingers are. Some nurses say this can't happen. Maybe not to them yet, but I have seen it happen. Call it a fluke or an accident, but remember, accidents can and will happen. Never place yourself in that precarious position.

Also, as you get ready to stick your patient, you want to always prepare them by telling them they will feel a *pinch* or a *stick*. You think your patients are ready, and *they* say they are, but once you puncture their skin with the needle, oftentimes patients jump, tense up, or pull back, which can cause you to miss your mark and give yourself a dirty needle stick. At other times, as you may be fishing around for the vein (especially with those who have very thin skin), you can go through the skin and give yourself a dirty needle stick. Therefore, drawing traction above the stick site is risky and just bad form.

Point number two. Stabilization is not truly achieved by drawing the vein in the proximal direction (upward toward the elbow). By drawing traction proximally and also inserting the needle in the proximal direction, you can cause the vein to bunch up and actually slacken, if you will, which makes for a difficult entry. Since the vein may actually loosen distally while applying proximal traction, you inherently lose stabilization, and may actually have to alter your angle of entry or may have to fish for the vein. This could cause you to go through the other side and blow the vein.

Drawing traction distally is the most effective way to achieve stabilization. Most clinicians will draw down on the skin, and their technique looks good, but it is usually not with enough force and downward pressure to stabilize the vein properly. To be effective and create the optimum chance of success, you need to apply *very firm*, let me repeat, *very firm,* downward pressure to truly stabilize the vein. So, you can apply traction, or you can apply *traction*.

There is more to this than just distal stretching of the skin and underlying vein, however. Many clinicians will apply *downward* or distal stretch by pulling straight down, but by doing so, they unknowingly obstruct the entry of their needle because they have to compete with their thumb when they get ready to stick. This only complicates the procedure. (Remember, comfort is everything, and having your thumb in the way will impinge on your comfort to insert the needle and advance the catheter.) The entry will also be at too steep of an angle, and you again run the risk of going through the vein. You have to get the thumb of your nondominant hand (your traction hand) out of the way. Therefore, the downward and outward traction technique is imperative and ideal for achieving success.

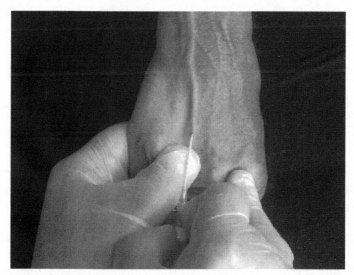

Wrong Traction: This is the wrong way to apply and hold traction. Notice how traction is straight downward and how the thumb of the nondominant hand gets in the way. Competing with the thumb forces you to alter your entry and go in at too steep of an angle. (BD Insyte™ Autoguard ™ IV catheter shown courtesy of Becton, Dickinson and Company)

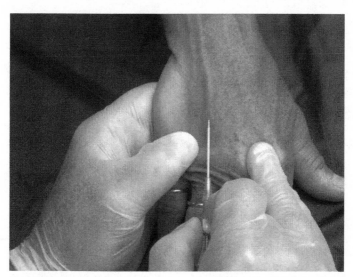

Proper Traction: Notice the proper way to apply downward and outward traction for proper stabilization of the vein. Notice how the thumb is now off to the side and entry to the vein can be made at a lower angle. (BD Insyte™ Autoguard ™ IV catheter shown courtesy of Becton, Dickinson and Company)

Keep your eye on the target:

Once you begin to apply traction, never take your eye off the prize. Starting an IV is like shooting hoops, pitching horseshoes, or target shooting. If you line up your shot or zero in on the target, your accuracy continues to improve. If you are distracted or take your eye off the target in any way prior to the stick (even for a moment), chances are you will miss, or at the very least, struggle with the IV. If you always watch your target as you apply traction, you will most often hit the vein on your first try. As traction is applied, there is always a small shift of the vein because you are purposefully stretching the skin to get your thumb out of the way. *You have to watch this shift.* This is very important. Over time, you will get better and better and more confident. Proper traction on the vein is essential; but remember, it must be *very firm traction.*

Stabilize the stick:

Applying traction to the vein is vital, but equally important and essential is stabilization of the stick. You must also have true stabilization and control of the needle/catheter device. I have seen many nurses try to start an IV with no control whatsoever of their needle. As they try to stick and think they are in control, many times their hand is basically free-floating. I have witnessed others rest on their knuckles (hard to imagine, isn't it?), but this limits their freedom of movement and control. Then, there are those who use three fingers to hold the catheter/needle device. They use their thumb and middle finger to hold the needle, while using their index finger to secure the catheter at the twelve o'clock position. This positioning is unnatural and uncomfortable, as your wrist is too flat and your hand is horizontal or parallel to the patient's arm. This is an improper entry plane to allow easy access. This, to me, is impractical because you cannot effectively pivot your hand to find your entry point. Don't take my word for it—try it.

Consider how your hand rests at the side of your body. Think of the position of your hand and wrist when you pick up a coffee cup or when you write with a pen? If you notice the subtlety of the movement, your wrist and hand most often face inward or medially to the body. This is the natural and most comfortable position for the hand and wrist. Therefore, when you hold your needle/catheter device, you should try to achieve this natural position for maximum success.

To achieve proper stabilization of the stick, all five fingers of your dominant hand are used. Your index finger holds the needle/catheter at the two o'clock position (ten o'clock position for left hand dominant), while your thumb and third (middle) finger stabilize the device. The fourth and fifth (pinky) fingers are used to act as a pivot point to provide control of the needle device. By pivoting off of your fourth and fifth fingers (mostly off of your fourth finger), you put your hand and wrist in the more natural medial (thirty-to-forty-five degree estimate) position. When you then steady your dominant hand, you have very fine micro-control and can easily direct where your needle is going.

One other key point to note—and this is important—as you go to stabilize your stick and plant your fourth and fifth fingers down as a pivot point, use these fingers to *lightly* stretch the patient's skin in the opposite direction; similar to your *downward and away* traction provided by your nondominant hand. You are now providing downward and away stretching or traction on the vein, both to the right and to the left, or medially and laterally below your proposed insertion point. This is very similar to the anchoring and stability of the bifurcated vein. In essence, you are triangulating the vein, if you will, for a more stable entry.

Finesse is everything. This is like using the fine adjustment on a microscope. Going for the stick is using the coarse adjustment, but going for the stick by using your other fingers as a pivot point and positioning you hand/wrist in a more natural position, is the fine adjustment or fine tuning of the technique.

Pulling distal downward and outward traction, keeping your eye on the target, and stabilizing the stick by using your fingers as a pivot are key elements to achieving success in initiating an IV. Remember, you need to put all components together. Stabilize the vein, stabilize the catheter (as we discussed earlier), and stabilize the stick.

Putting It All Together—
Going for the Stick

Unless you are in an emergent situation and need a *quick stick* right away, what's the rush? I cannot stress this enough. Slow down; take your time. I have heard some say that a *quick stick* is less painful and traumatizing to the patient. This may be appropriate at times in an emergency, but the best way to achieve success is to slow down. You need to be meticulous. You need to be like a jeweler cutting a diamond. You have to be totally focused and engaged as you perform your actions (getting relaxed, drawing very tight traction, achieving total stabilization, and making a slow entry into the vein).

Now that we have discussed the subtleties of what to look for, you are ready to stick the vein. One key element to take into account each and every time is the design of your over the needle/catheter device. Many clinicians take this for granted, but if you observe how the catheter fits over the needle, always remember that it sits behind the bevel of the needle. The catheter sits about one-to-two millimeters behind the sharp point of the needle (depending on the catheter size), as we discussed earlier. It is important to know this because it impacts what happens after you get flashback.

Now, here's some information on flashback. Flashback is the occurrence of blood entering the catheter and collection chamber of the needle device once the vein is punctured. Quite often, nurses and paramedics note flashback as blood traveling up the catheter into the space between the catheter and needle. This is an indication that you probably did hit the vein, but it can give you a false sense of security. It is not a confirmation that you are in the vein. It has happened to me many times; I get a little bit of blood into the catheter, but I cannot advance the catheter. These times, I believe I really just nicked the vein while searching for it, and then I probably pulled out of the vein prematurely.

The only way to know that you are in the vein is to assure that you get flashback (blood) all the way up to the collection chamber of the over the needle device. I have started many IVs and have blown the vein because I only saw the blood running up the catheter, thinking I was in the vein. I never looked at the collection chamber. Conversely, I have tried to initiate many IVs where I never saw flashback coming up the catheter, and as I fished around, I became frustrated and withdrew my needle, only to realize that I had blood in the collection chamber and was in the vein all along. My problem was that I never looked at the flash chamber because I was only concentrating on flashback coming up the catheter. Don't fall into this trap the way I did. As you are initiating your IV and think, *I've got to be in the vein,"* always glance at the collection chamber. You need to have blood there to be sure you have hit the vein properly.

Some of you may say, *I've stuck my patient, and I am sure I have to be in the vein, but I did not get any flashback.* This same phenomenon has happened to me on several occasions. There are sometimes exceptions to the rule. Your vein is right there, and you are positive you have to be in the vein, but never get any flashback.

In my experience, sometimes you have to stop where you are with your stick, and just wait several seconds. I know this is a hard concept to accept. You might even think I'm crazy, but I have learned enough times that this is a very real phenomenon. When it happens, sometimes I will release the tourniquet, and blood will slowly begin to come into the catheter. At that point, I resume my advance and many times have saved the IV.

I really don't have an explanation for why this happens, but sometimes just pausing and waiting several seconds allows the blood of low pressure patients to slowly enter the needle/catheter device. Remember, however, you always must get blood back before you can claim that the IV is patent and useable. Also remember, you have to be meticulous and focused, just like a jeweler cutting a diamond. Don't get discouraged.

As you begin to stick, inform patients they will feel *a stick* or *a pinch* or whatever verbiage you want to use, but most of all, encourage them to relax. Putting patients at ease is critical. How many times have you tried an IV, only to have the patient tense up and pull away? Once the patient tenses his hand or arm, the muscles under the skin can form around the vein and can cause the vein to shift away from your planned insertion point, even if you are holding proper traction.

Once I sense the patient tightening up, I begin talking to them with urgency, encouraging them to *relax, relax, relax. Don't tighten your hand. Relax, relax; you need to relax.* They usually get the message, and you can sense when they start to relax and loosen up their hand or arm. At that point, I often advance my stick and get the IV. This works almost every time; it all boils down to *them* sensing *your* confidence and *you* putting *them* at ease.

As you begin to puncture the skin (remember to secure or stabilize your catheter for a slow entry into the vein), always make sure the bevel of the needle is facing up, and be sure to keep a low profile.

A low profile approach to the vein is best—perhaps at a fifteen degree or less angle. Going in at too steep of an angle is unstable (remember that you have to stabilize the stick), and you run the risk of puncturing through the other end of the vein. You do not want to go in at too steep of an angle.

I know a career hemodialysis nurse who took a job at the bedside and was having difficulty initiating IVs. She was always able to access her patient's fistulas or shunts, and she said she never had a problem before. When we went over all of the techniques (included in this book), she realized that she was using too steep of an angle to stick for a peripheral IV. She told me later that, when accessing a dialysis patient's shunt or fistula, you need to go in at a steep angle because their access is deep, but she also realized when starting a basic peripheral IV on a patient, you need a low profile to be successful. It took this great nurse some adjustment to get used to it, but now she is more confident and successful.

When you get flashback into the collection chamber of the over the needle catheter device, it is an indication that the needle has entered the vein. However, if you observe Illustration 3—Figure A, you can see *it is very possible to get flashback and not have the catheter fully inserted into the vein.* If this is the case and you don't realize it, you may have a false sense of security, thinking you are fully into the vein, and in turn, you will never be able to advance the catheter. You will then *blow* the vein. Getting flashback is not a guarantee that your catheter is in the vein, but most new nurses think so and will still try to slide the catheter in. That is when problems arise.

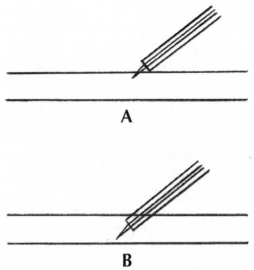

Illustration 3—Flashback can be obtained with just the bevel of the needle in the vein (Figure A). Be sure to insert the needle catheter device two-to-three millimeters more to insure the catheter is in the vein (Figure B).

Probably the most vital step and key to success is that when you get initial flashback, you need to just *pause for a moment*, and at this point, lower the needle toward the skin to reduce the angle even more. Your needle is now almost parallel to the skin. Think about the direction of the vein, and keep your eye on the prize. (Remember, you are still holding traction.)

Once you do this, *you have to advance your needle/catheter device into the vein about two-to-three millimeters more to insure the catheter is truly in the vein*, as indicated in Illustration 3—Figure B. (Remember your needle/catheter design and how the catheter sits roughly about one millimeter behind the bevel for the smallest catheter size (24 gauge), while the catheter is a little more than two millimeters for the larger (16 gauge) catheter. Do this very slowly, especially with diabetics and geriatric patients. It's all about poise and finesse. *This is a critical juncture for success and is probably the single most important step needed to be consistently successful.*

Two-to-three millimeters is not a lot. It doesn't take much. I cannot stress enough how important this step is. Most people think they know what two-to-three millimeters looks like, but in reality, I have found that they really don't. They usually overestimate its length. Do you know how much two-to-three millimeters really is? Do you know what it looks like?

Take a look at the characters below.

--

Those two dashes are roughly two millimeters in length. Doesn't look like much, does it? The thickness of a quarter is roughly this size. So freeze these images in your mind, and keep perspective when initiating an IV. Once you get flashback, you only have to advance just that much more to insure the catheter is in the vein. Take your macro thinking almost to the micro level. This will help improve your success rate tremendously.

I have seen nurses advance the catheter way too far in most cases. I estimate some to be almost one whole centimeter (that's three to five times too much), and many a good IV has been blown this way. *In the world of IVs, less is better.* You are advancing by micro-amounts, if you will. Two-to-three millimeters does not look like a lot, but usually it is plenty to insure entry of the plastic catheter into the vein.

To repeat the critical point, once you get flashback, you have to slow everything down, pause, lower your needle to the skin surface, and then make your advance into the vein by two-to-three millimeters. (I may sometimes only advance by one-to-two millimeters, depending on the patient.) You have to advance by this amount to clear the thickness of the vessel wall and insure the catheter is truly in the vein. This advancement of the catheter into the vein is paramount to being successful at initiating good sound IVs. Keep in mind, however, that as you advance *ever so slightly,* you need to follow the track of the vein.

As you can see, all of this requires fine dexterity and poise.

Two-handed catheter advance:

Once I know the catheter is in the vein, I can release the traction from my nondominant hand and slide the catheter up into the vein. I must tell you that I am not an advocate of the single-finger advance technique. This is where, after getting into the vein, the clinician continues to maintain traction on the vein, while attempting to advance the catheter by using the index finger of the dominant hand that is holding the over the needle catheter device. I see nurses do this, or attempt to do this, all the time, and many times, they are unsuccessful and quite often, break asepsis.

I *have* seen the one finger advance work on occasion, but that is when you have the perfect patient with nice big veins. In our world of medicine, however, we most often will never see the perfect patient because our patients are ill. I honestly feel that the one finger advance is just too risky.

Observing other clinicians closely as they attempt this technique, several things happen. Some nurses hold the needle with their thumb and index finger to start the IV; then, as they advance the catheter, they switch to holding the device with their thumb and third finger to free up their index finger to advance the catheter. By doing this, the angle of the needle is changed ever so slightly and makes it more difficult for the catheter to enter or advance up the vein. This is an unstable approach.

Second, by trying to advance the catheter with the index finger, the pivot point for stabilizing the hand changes and the dominant hand is no longer secure or stable. (Remember, you have to stabilize the vein and stabilize the stick.) This being the case, as the clinician tries to advance the catheter (with the single finger technique), he or she unknowingly pushes or rocks the needle back and forth (in micro increments), which can cause the point of the needle to puncture the intima or other side of the vein. Then when the clinician tries to advance the catheter, he or she is unable to do so.

Third, by using the tip of the index finger to slide the catheter forward, many times the nurse does not use the slide notch on the hub; remember, we turned the catheter a quarter turn to loosen it. Therefore, the nurse usually pushes the catheter forward using the end of the hub where the extension set or IV line will be connected, and quite often, can break asepsis and contaminate the hub end and put the patient at risk.

I advocate using the two-handed technique. God gave us two hands; why not use them? This is very similar to the phlebotomist who accesses a blood draw, and once inside the vein, stabilizes the needle so that it doesn't move. He/she then uses the other hand to interchange her blood tubes, again, never moving the needle.

Once I am sure the catheter is in the vein (after my two-to-three millimeter advance), I can let go of my traction. I have not let go of my over the needle catheter device, however, and have not changed my pivot or stabilizing point. My needle is solid, steady, and secure—again, similar to a phlebotomist drawing blood. I then reach over with my nondominant hand, use my thumb and index finger of this hand to grab the outside of the hub, and advance the catheter. All the while, I'm observing the puncture point and watching for any problems or complications as I guide the catheter into the vein. Never lose sight of your insertion point.

Floating the catheter in:

At the slightest sign of difficulty or if the catheter does not slide easily into the vein and you meet resistance, *do not force it*. Difficulty advancing the catheter can be caused by being up against a valve, a sclerotic vein, or the vein being squiggly or wavy. If you get overly aggressive and try to force the catheter, you will quite often go through the vein and blow it. You need to slow everything down.

Trying to advance the catheter past a valve or up a wavy vein to make it patent; this is what we call *floating the catheter in*. To do this, first tamponade (apply proximal pressure to compress the vein and prevent blood leakage from the catheter hub) above the insertion site (where you think the tip of the catheter is located) before you remove the needle (from inside the catheter). It is very important that when you tamponade, you also secure the hub of the catheter so it does not slip out of the vein. I usually use the fourth finger of my nondominant hand to tamponade, while using my thumb and index finger to grab and hold the catheter hub.

Next, maintain strict asepsis, and by using your dominant hand, hook up your primed extension tubing with a sterile saline syringe already attached. Prior to doing this, I sometimes slip a 2x2 gauze pad under the hub of the catheter to catch any blood leakage. Be sure your connection is tight, or you can leak at this connection. You can now release hold of the catheter hub from your nondominant hand since you are now holding the catheter/tubing connection with your dominant hand. You are now ready to float the catheter in. At this point, I will firmly tell my patient, *don't move!*

Give small pulsations of sterile saline using your nondominant hand, and at the same time, turn and roll the catheter hub (as if you are rolling a pencil between your thumb and index finger), while *gently* advancing the catheter in. You need to roll and gently push or advance the catheter inward all at the same time.

Basically the *floating* technique is *pulse and push*, pulse and push. Remember, *pulse with saline, and roll and push the catheter. Pulse and push.*

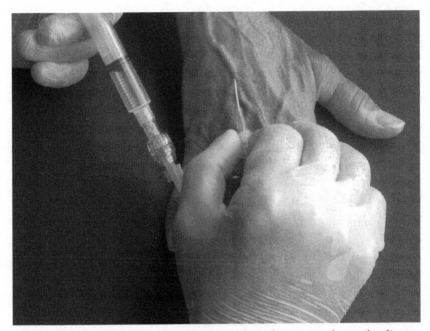

Floating the catheter in: Notice when floating in the catheter, you pulse sterile saline using your nondominant hand, while rolling the threaded connector/hub forward with your dominant hand. All the while, you are advancing the catheter into the vein. (ONE-LINK Needle-free Connector and extension set shown with permission by Baxter Healthcare Corporation. Baxter is a trademark of Baxter International Inc., All rights reserved. BD Insyte™ Autoguard ™ IV catheter shown courtesy of Becton, Dickinson and Company)

Don't misunderstand when I use the word *push*, however, because it is more like a gentle coring of the vein to slide the catheter up into the lumen. The goal is to advance the catheter all the way up to the hub. Remember to maintain good aseptic technique, as you do not want to contaminate the puncture site.

Be sure to constantly check for infiltration above the insertion site while you are flushing with your sterile saline. You will notice an infiltrated site because the skin will have localized swelling where the end of the catheter rests under the skin. A patent IV should always have good blood return and lack any localized swelling.

Rarely, but occasionally, you may notice some minor bruising at the site. This may occur with elderly patients and sometimes with those on anticoagulation. This does not mean the site is necessarily bad or unusable. If you were able to advance the catheter and still have a good blood return, you are probably okay. The rule of thumb however is that if you feel uncomfortable with the site at all, pull the IV and start over in a different location.

Now that your IV has been successfully established, *always* remember to release your tourniquet either before you begin taping or after you secure the site. This is a personal preference. However, failure to do this can cause serious harm to your patient. In addition, if you should stick the site but by chance miss the IV, again, you *must* remember to remove the tourniquet.

Fragile Veins—Diabetic and Geriatric Patients:

Be very careful when trying to initiate an IV on diabetic or geriatric patients. These types of patients have extremely fragile veins, plus many geriatric (and renal) patients have extremely thin skin, causing their veins to be very *surface oriented*.

Diabetics:

To be perfectly honest, diabetic veins are difficult to access, primarily because they are extremely delicate and flimsy, not to mention thin and narrow. It is not within the scope of this book to discuss the pathophysiology of how and why this occurs with diabetics, but instead to make you aware that your skill really comes into play here.

I once cared for a lifelong diabetic patient who appeared to have decent veins. No problem, right? Wrong! I stuck for a hand vein, and it totally disappeared. I fished around for it and nicked it, but no matter how much I tried to hit it, I couldn't get into the vein. Next, I went for a nice looking forearm vein. I got a good flashback and advanced without difficulty. Once I withdrew my needle, I still got blood up into the catheter. No problem, right? Wrong! I released the tourniquet, and as soon as I flushed to verify patency, the vein blew. The patient ended up with a hard knot above the insertion site, and I had to pull the IV.

I then asked another nurse (an excellent one and a good friend), who is extremely proficient at initiating IVs, to come look and try to obtain access. He looked and stuck, and the IV blew. Again, he found a nice vein, got great flashback, and had no problem with the advance, but as soon as he attempted to flush for patency, the IV blew. We were both confounded as to why our IVs were infiltrating. Finally, my friend suggested sticking without using a tourniquet. We held our breath and finally got the IV. My good friend applied some minor proximal pressure with his hands, and we were able to get good flashback, advance, and flush without blowing the vein. So much for the one-and-done! This just goes to show you how truly fragile this man's veins were. Even using a looser tourniquet did not help our cause.

The point is that diabetic veins are different, and you can't take anything for granted. Be cautious, be careful, and be smart when starting IVs on a diabetic, but don't shy away from it. Remember, you are the one that got the IV. That is the takeaway.

Geriatric Patients:

Geriatric patients usually have very thin skin. Their veins run close to the surface of the skin, and it doesn't take much to go right through them if you are too aggressive. I have found that when initiating an IV on these patients, you really need to slow down your approach and stick. You must avoid, at all cost, being too aggressive. Go very, very slowly.

Quite often, you may just barely start your stick, when you suddenly get immediate flashback. It is truly surprising and almost unfathomable how close to the skin surface their veins can be. It is at this point that you really need to pause for a moment and then, ever so slightly—I repeat—ever so slightly, advance your needle/catheter device maybe one-to-two millimeters (not the recommended two-to-three millimeters, as stated earlier). These patients' veins must always be approached with reservation and caution, and you need to always respect how fragile their veins can be. Again, this is where your poise and professionalism will really be put to the test.

Most often I find with diabetic and geriatric veins that it is best not to try to advance the catheter all the way in but to cautiously float it in, and certainly you do not want to force the catheter. I have tried many times to advance the catheter all the way in on these types of patients, never meeting resistance, only to find I went right through the vein and infiltrated with my flush. Talk about frustration! I thought it was good, and everything looked good, only to find I blew the vein. So the lesson is, do not take anything for granted when you have diabetic, geriatric, or even renal patients. Sometimes the rules change; often you need to adapt, but always, you need to utilize extra care and caution.

One last thing is that you may want or need to try the next smaller size catheter than what you first anticipated. Remember, that's okay. Many times with these patients, it is more important to get the lifeline than to worry about the size of the catheter.

Believe in yourself. You can do it. I know you can.

Secure and Tape the Site

Now that the catheter is in and the extension set is attached, it is time to secure the IV. For many years (and the way I learned to tape an IV in place) it has been common practice to use the *Chevron* taping method. This is where you take a thin piece of tape about two-to-three inches long and about one-quarter inch or less wide, and slip it under the hub of the catheter, crisscrossing the ends over the top of the hub. You then tape over this piece of tape or apply the clear occlusive dressing over the hub. This method is still being taught and has been the so-called standard taping procedure for decades. This has not been my standard, however.

This is a very inefficient taping method. If you think about it, when lifting the catheter hub to slip your Chevron tape underneath, if you are not paying attention to detail, it is easy to dislodge the catheter because you are moving it back and forth and up and down. Quite often the nurse is focused on the taping rather than what is happening to the catheter. Also, it is reasonable to assume that this movement can and does cause damage to the intima or inner lining of the vessel.

I find the other significant thing wrong with the Chevron method is that it is a loose taping job at best and does not firmly secure the catheter in place. (I can only assume that it was first introduced to create forward pull on the catheter hub to maintain and secure the catheter into the puncture site.) Truthfully, it does not work and is not beneficial for longevity of the IV. Also, if you have to re-dress the site for any reason, it is a very frustrating experience, as you will have to undo the Chevron tape and can quite often accidently pull out the IV. It's happened to me. *My advice: don't Chevron.*

When I was a rookie paramedic, I was on an emergency call one day; my patient was becoming more and more critically ill right before my eyes. As I stated earlier, I, too, learned to Chevron my IVs (just like everyone else), and after initiating one on my patient, there I was trying to secure the IV *properly* with the Chevron. I guess I wanted to be a good paramedic, and I was under-exposed to the world of EMS. As my patient kept deteriorating, I was fumbling around to try not to lose the IV. I realized my patient was getting worse and said to myself, *The heck with it*, and proceeded to just take tape and secure it the best way I could. We had to move and get this patient to the hospital. At that time, it was drilled into all of us that we had to Chevron to secure the IV prop-erly. I was only trying to do what I was trained to do, but I was also very naive.

Now everyone knows that paramedics are trained to think outside the box, but that you also follow your training and protocols to the tee. The more I thought about it, I saw how inefficient the Chevron taping method was. What I did that day was use three pieces of tape. I have been taping my IVs that way ever since, and my taping method has never failed me. I stand it up to anyone's for security and safety of the IV.

When I became a nurse and started taping *my way*, I was informed by a number of nurses in our unit that *we can't tape that way*. I was told that I would be *talked to* about *proper taping of IVs* using the Chevron method. Well, I was never challenged. Now when I teach how to properly tape an IV, I teach nurses and other clinicians my way. You may think this is a menial, insignificant point to make, and that it is no big deal, or ask why am I devoting so much time on taping of an IV?

The important thing is that after you become proficient at initiating IVs (and you will), that is only half the battle. What good is it to become good at starting IVs if you can't secure the site properly, and you run the risk of losing it? *It is essential to tape properly.*

Another poor taping technique I've seen is when the clinician puts the occlusive dressing over both the hub and screw connection together. I find this to be a problem, as too much of a gap exists under the catheter hub result-ing in an ineffective dressing. Also, the catheter is not secure and can easily become dislodged over a short period of time. My advice is to avoid this pitfall as well. I know the occlusive dressing's purpose is to maintain asepsis to the puncture site, but if applied properly, it can also help secure the IV catheter.

To more effectively secure an IV, you need only the occlusive dressing and three pieces of tape about four inches long. Once the extension set has been attached and screwed on, the first step is to place a piece of tape over the threaded connector only. This holds the IV in place. Next, the occlusive dressing should *abut* up to the threaded connection, but not be placed over it, so that it only covers the hub of the catheter. This, if properly applied, is what secures the catheter in place and protects the puncture site.

Next, make a small loop with the extension set, and place your second piece of tape directly over the first piece, securing the loop of the extension set. Lastly, at the distal end of the extension where your needleless connector is, place the last piece of tape.

I make every effort not to put any tape over the occlusive dressing because the tape has aggressive adhesion and is difficult to remove if needed; sometimes this is unavoidable. Your IV should now be nicely secure, and fear of losing it is minimal at best. You may now think that what I just described is simple and just common sense, but I can tell you that most practitioners do not apply it. I am all for common sense—not for fancy taping.

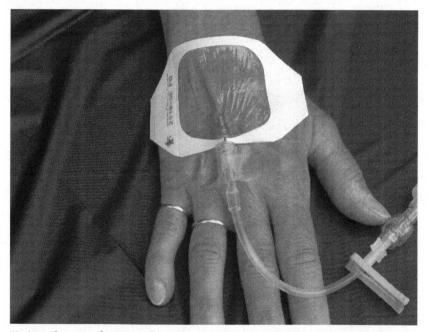

Taping: Place your first piece of tape over the extension tubing threaded connector after inserting and securing it to the IV catheter hub. Notice how the occlusive dressing is only placed over the catheter hub to secure it. Do not cover the threaded connector with the occlusive dressing. (ONE-LINK Needle-free IV connector and extension set shown with permission by Baxter Healthcare Corporation. Baxter is a trademark of Baxter International Inc., All rights reserved. BD Insyte™ Autoguard ™ IV catheter shown courtesy of Becton, Dickinson and Company. IV start kit supplies and Tegaderm (trademark of 3M Company) occlusive dressing shown are from Medline Industries Inc. "IV Start Kit" courtesy of Medline Industries, Inc.)

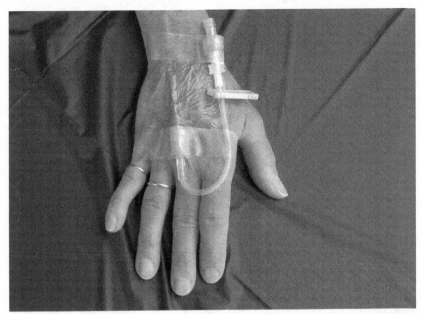

Securely taped IV: The picture above shows a totally secure IV with the suggested taping method. You may have to improvise and vary your taping depending on the IV's location. (ONE-LINK Needle-free IV connector and extension tubing shown with permission by Baxter Healthcare Corporation. Baxter is a trademark of Baxter International Inc., All rights reserved. BD Insyte™ Autoguard ™ IV catheter shown courtesy of Becton, Dickinson and Company. IV start kit supplies and Tegaderm (trademark of 3M Company) occlusive dressing shown are from Medline Industries Inc. "IV Start Kit" courtesy of Medline Industries, Inc.)

Again, IV taping is like tying your shoes. The more you do it, the better you become at it. Remember, there is less movement to the catheter, less damage to the intima of the vessel, and the site is more secure—no Chevron used and no loose taping.

Another benefit is that if blood leaks beneath the occlusive dressing and you need to change it, you can do this easily by just removing the occlusive dressing alone or with only one piece of tape, keeping the other two pieces of tape in place and protecting the extension tubing/hub connection. The IV remains secure, and you minimize the risk of losing it if you had Chevroned.

Also, if you do have to re-tape your patient's IV, you can keep the occlusive dressing in place, and just re-do the taping portion. There are benefits all around, so proper taping is imperative to initiate and maintain a successful IV. Most of your IVs can be taped this way, but sometimes you have to get creative due to the location of the IV. Experiment with this. Imagination is the mother of invention.

If your patient is in shock and very diaphoretic, and the tape is not sticking, you may have to wrap the site with roller gauze or even use an elastic self-adherent wrap such as Coban (trademark of 3M Company). Remember though, that when you wrap the site, you need to wrap it so that you can always view the catheter insertion site.

Check your site for leakage or infiltration a minimum of every four hours or more frequently if needed to insure patency of the IV. You never want to assume everything is okay. Always have a high index of suspicion, even when you think the IV is good. You need to consider the integrity of the patient's veins (old veins, diabetic veins, etc.). Also, as in the ICU, many very harsh medicines are used to regulate blood pressure or cardiac dysrhythmias. These can break down fragile veins quickly, so be vigilant and check your IV sites routinely. Always adhere to your medical organization's IV protocol.

Sometimes Two Is Better

Initiating an IV is usually a one-man job, and we all take pride in getting the *difficult stick*. We will do anything to prove our worth because most of us have something to prove to ourselves. We are human beings, and many times pride gets in the way. If we can't get the IV, we feel embarrassed and worry about how we are viewed by others. Do they think of us as inadequate or incompetent? (I have been there. Remember, I'm the guy who had fifteen misses in a row.) These are certainly natural feelings to have, but we have to put pride aside.

There is nothing wrong in asking one of your colleagues to assist if necessary. Sometimes two is better. The geriatric population usually has very loose skin, and often, their veins roll. These veins frequently cannot be secured properly, even with good proper downward and away traction because the skin is too loose.

What I have done in these circumstances is to ask another nurse to stretch the skin horizontally or medially and laterally on the arm/hand to remove the *skin factor*. This action now better exposes the vein and decreases the *roll factor*. With my partner in place stretching the skin, I can now pull my downward and away traction to optimize stabilization of the vein. When you make your stick, you have increased you chances of establishing a successful IV.

You can also ask a colleague to hold and rotate a patient's arm for maximum access. This allows you better visibility and comfort, and you don't have to wrestle with the patient to steady the access point.

Lesson to learn: don't be afraid to ask for assistance. We are all in this together, and remember, our ultimate goal is the security and safety of the patient. Do no harm. Get the IV on the first attempt. *One and done* is the goal.

Labeling and Documentation

Now that the IV is established and taped, it is important to label the site. All IVs should be labeled with the date and time established, the size catheter used, and the name of the person initiating the IV. Many times, the labels that come in start packs do not adhere well to tape, so I usually apply another piece of tape over the label to secure it. This enhances longevity of the label, making it easy for any clinician to track its age. A piece of tape over the label also protects it from moisture damage when bathing a patient.

I usually place my label over the pieces of tape, securing the threaded connector of the extension set, but anywhere you choose is acceptable. Again, I try not to place anything sticky (like tape or labels) over the transparent occlusive dressing, as these are difficult to remove if re-taping is needed. Quite often, trying to remove tape on the occlusive dressing also pulls up the dressing; then your whole site needs to be re-dressed.

After all is said and done, the last item that needs to be done is proper documentation. It is imperative to do this honestly and correctly. It goes without saying that the type of access (peripheral IV) needs to be defined, along with your name, date, time, site, and size of the catheter.

A statement should always be included indicating that *aseptic technique* was properly used. This is no different than when a surgeon dictates in his procedure notes a statement indicating his surgical site was prepped in the *usual sterile fashion.*

The important thing here is that if you are initiating the IV, you need to be proficient and confident that your aseptic technique is excellent. You cannot use this statement if you have poor technique. That would be false. Your integrity and character are at stake here. Remember, using proper, strict aseptic technique insures the safety of the patient. Refer back to the earlier chapter on asepsis and reference about scrubbing the site vigorously and avoiding re-touching the site to re-palpate the vein. These steps are critical to proper technique.

Once you have established that proper aseptic technique was used, how can you define in your charting that the IV is functional and patent? Most nurses will usually include a statement that the IV *flushes without difficulty* or *no infiltration is noted* when flushing with sterile saline solution. This does not appropriately indicate a good, patent IV.

What if your patient is morbidly obese? I challenge you to realistically state with all certainty that the IV is patent because you did not see signs of infiltration under the skin. Most IV flushes are five-to-ten milliliters of sterile saline. Isn't it entirely possible the sterile saline could have flushed under the skin of a morbidly obese person, and you could not detect an infiltration?

The only way to properly state that your IV is patent is if you include a statement to the effect that a *good blood return* was obtained and that the IV *flushes without difficulty*. Again, this *must* be a truthful statement on your part. If you are not sure of the patency of your IV, remove it. *Rule of thumb: When in doubt, take it out.* As a nurse or other healthcare clinician, you have to advocate for your patient and do no harm. You should always have your patient's best interest at heart. No one cares about your ego.

Conclusion

Initiating a peripheral intravenous line is a skill that needs to be appropriately honed by the respective nurse, paramedic, or advanced clinician. As with anything else in life, this technique is not as easy as it looks. Sure, you can watch someone do it many times and think it looks easy enough, but only when you try it yourself will you realize some of the difficulties involved. Not everyone has big, bulging veins. Many fine points (that most people never even think about) should be considered before you even go for the initial stick.

As a new nurse or paramedic, you may get a taste of success and feel pretty good about yourself. As an experienced nurse or paramedic, you have already been on the front lines. Each and every IV success is a new victory and needs to be celebrated, but don't get too comfortable with yourself because your next miss is only your next IV away.

Every patient is different, and every approach may vary, but consistency is what you want to achieve. You want to be excellent at what you do and increase your success rate. That comes with practice, paying attention to detail, not getting overly confident with yourself, and not shying away from the difficult stick. You should always be prepared for the challenge.

To get really good at this most fundamental nursing and paramedic skill, you must pay attention to the details. Honing the fine points will take you from being average and craft you into being excellent. Believe me, your patient will appreciate you, and you will become more confident in your own abilities. Remember the one and done rule. That is the approach you want to take.

Many years ago, I found myself at the rock-bottom of the barrel. My confidence was gone, and I questioned what I was doing caring for patients when I couldn't even give them one of the most important interventions they needed to get well. It was only through analyzing my approach that I was able to become more proficient at initiating the peripheral intravenous line. These techniques and tricks work for me, and I firmly believe they will work for you, too. You not only have to apply them, but you also have to develop your own style or finesse. Develop your own *art*.

My hope is that, by following some or all of the suggestions in this book, you, too, will become more proficient, and your confidence will soar. I know it will. You can do it! Never give up on yourself. *Your patients depend upon you.*

Appendix

Key steps to remember when initiating a peripheral intravenous line:

1) Always practice universal precautions.
2) Develop excellent aseptic technique.
3) Use tight-fitting gloves.
4) Know your landmarks.
5) Tourniquet above the elbow.
6) After finding the vein you want, release the tourniquet to relieve pressure (unless emergent).
7) Start low and work high.
8) *Go for the Bifurcate.*
9) Mark the site (fingernail mark).
10) Prepare your extension tubing and set yourself up.
11) Loosen the catheter only a quarter turn. Never slide up and down on the needle.
12) *Secure the catheter.*
13) *Secure the site.* Always apply *very firm traction.*
14) *Secure the stick.*
15) Follow the shift. (When you draw traction, don't take your eye off the target.)
16) Use a low-profile approach.
17) Bevel up. Once you get flashback, lower your angle to the skin even more.
18) *Advance the catheter 2-3 mm into the vein after getting flashback.*
19) Avoid the one-finger advance.
20) Avoid the Chevron.
21) Sometimes two is better.

22) *When in doubt, take it out.*
23) Document properly.
24) *Relax and be confident. You are better than you think. You just don't know it yet.*

Best of luck to you on your future successes!

Acknowledgments

None of us ever gets through life without having to rely on someone else. We are all in this together. Those that have helped me achieve the goal of writing this book are special. This book is written with special thanks to:

God, who guides my hand and my heart.

My wife, Terry, you are my rock. Your constant encouragement and belief in me are humbling. I love you so very much.

My son, Paul, your zest for life is inspiring and a beautiful thing to watch. Your willingness to learn will allow you to achieve great things. Never stop learning. Thanks for helping with the photos in this book.

My son, David, you have been my inspiration since you were a young boy. I've seen you achieve many great goals, and the sky is the limit for you to reach your dream. Thank you, also, for assisting with the photos in this book.

Heather Fryzlewicz, for your assistance with the photographs for this book. Thank you for your valued insights.

Dr. Dave Arnold, for your encouragement and support in writing this book. The completion of *your* book ignited a fire in me to write mine. We never know how what we say or do will affect others. Your positive inspiration has helped me to believe in myself.

Fred Antoun Jr., Esq., for your oversight in the preparation of this book. Thank you for all of your professional advice and legal expertise in helping me appreciate the ins and outs of the publishing industry. You are a very fine man and have become a good friend. Thank you for everything.

Fred Kuhn, President of LA Cameras in Chambersburg, PA. Your help in guiding me in the understanding of my camera and suggestions for obtaining picture quality were immeasurable.

Wendy Harrington, Stephanie McClure, and the editors and designers of Archway Publishing who have helped me navigate through the world of book publishing. More than I can say, I appreciate your unwavering commitment to excellence.

Karen Frey of Medline Industries, Inc., Judy Noah and Ryan Murphy of Baxter Healthcare Corp., and Dawn Harley, Matthew O'Connell, and David Myers of Becton, Dickinson and Company for the images and intravenous supplies and samples you supplied to help make this project complete. Thank you for your support.

Lastly, to Karla Seville RN, for allowing me access to your professional resources. *You* are a true professional. Thank you so very much.

43780676R00052

Made in the USA
Lexington, KY
12 August 2015